Everything You Need to
Know About Celiac Disease

Celiac disease is a chronic digestive and immune disorder that damages the small intestine. The disease is triggered by eating foods containing gluten. Gluten is a protein found naturally in wheat, barley, and rye, and is common in foods such as bread, pasta, cookies, and cakes. Many products contain gluten, such as prepackaged foods, lip balms and lipsticks, toothpastes, vitamin and nutrient supplements, and, rarely, medicines.

Celiac disease can be serious. The disease can cause long-lasting digestive problems and keep your body from getting all the nutrients it needs. Celiac disease can also affect the body outside the small intestine.

Celiac disease is different from gluten sensitivity or wheat intolerance. If you have gluten sensitivity, you may have symptoms like those of celiac disease, such as abdominal pain and tiredness. Unlike celiac disease, gluten sensitivity does not damage the small intestine.

Celiac disease is also different from a wheat allergy, a type of food allergy. In both cases, your body's immune system reacts to wheat. However, some symptoms of wheat allergies, such as having itchy eyes or a hard time breathing, are different from celiac disease. Wheat allergies also do not cause long-term damage to the small intestine.

Does celiac disease have other names?

Celiac disease is also called celiac sprue, nontropical sprue, and gluten-sensitive enteropathy.

How common is celiac disease?

Many people who have celiac disease have not been diagnosed. However, experts estimate about 2 million people in the United States have celiac disease and about 1 percent of people around the world have celiac disease.[1,2]

Who is more likely to develop celiac disease?

Celiac disease can only occur in people who have certain genes. You are more likely to develop celiac disease if someone in your family has the disease.

Celiac disease affects children and adults in all parts of the world. In the United States, celiac disease is more common among white Americans than among other racial or ethnic groups. A celiac disease diagnosis is more common in females than in males.[1]

Everything You Need to
Know About Celiac Disease

Causes ♦ Symptoms ♦ Treatment

Watch a video version:
https://www.youtube.com/watch?v=LkKWjmD1yeo

This book is based on information and recommendations by the Department of Health, United States government.

Created By The Bizmove Health Team

Disclaimer

All the content found in this book was created for informational purposes only. The Content is not intended to be a substitute for professional medical advice, diagnosis, or treatment. Always seek the advice of your physician or other qualified health provider with any questions you may have regarding a medical condition. Never disregard professional medical advice or delay in seeking it because of something you have read in this book.

Celiac disease is also more common in people who have certain chromosomal disorders, such as Down syndrome, Turner syndrome, and Williams syndrome.

What other health problems do people with celiac disease have?

Experts have found that some people have both celiac disease and other disorders related to the immune system. These disorders include

- type 1 diabetes
- thyroid diseases, such as Hashimoto's disease, Graves' disease, Addison's disease, and primary hyperparathyroidism
- selective immunoglobulin A (IgA) deficiency, a condition in which your body makes little or no IgA, an antibody that fights infections
- rheumatic diseases, such as Sjögren's syndrome
- liver diseases, such as autoimmune hepatitis, primary sclerosing cholangitis, and primary biliary cholangitis

What are the complications of celiac disease?

Long-term complications of celiac disease include

- accelerated osteoporosis or bone softening, known as osteomalacia
- anemia

- malnutrition, a condition in which you don't get enough vitamins, minerals, and other nutrients you need to be healthy
- nervous system problems
- problems related to the reproductive system

Rare complications can include

- adenocarcinoma, a type of cancer of the small intestine
- liver damage, which may lead to cirrhosis or liver failure
- non-Hodgkin lymphoma

In rare cases, you may continue to have trouble absorbing nutrients even though you have been following a strict gluten-free diet. If you have this condition, called refractory celiac disease, your small intestine is severely damaged and can't heal. You may need to receive intravenous (IV) nutrients and specialized treatment.

What are the symptoms of celiac disease?

Symptoms of celiac disease vary widely, and a person may have multiple symptoms that come and go. If you have celiac disease, you may have digestive problems or other symptoms. Digestive symptoms are more common in children than in adults. Digestive symptoms of celiac disease may include

- bloating
- chronic diarrhea
- constipation
- gas
- lactose intolerance due to damage to the small intestine
- loose, greasy, bulky, and bad-smelling stools
- nausea or vomiting
- pain in the abdomen

For children with celiac disease, being unable to absorb nutrients at a time when they are so important to normal growth and development can lead to

- damage to the permanent teeth's enamel
- delayed puberty
- failure to thrive, meaning that an infant or a child weighs less or is gaining less weight than expected for his or her age
- mood changes or feeling annoyed or impatient
- slowed growth and short height
- weight loss

Some people with celiac disease have symptoms that affect other parts of the body. These symptoms may include

- dermatitis herpetiformis
- fatigue, or feeling tired

- joint or bone pain
- mental health problems, such as depression or anxiety
- nervous system symptoms, such as headaches, balance problems, seizures, or peripheral neuropathy
- reproductive problems in women and girls—which may include infertility, delayed start of menstrual periods, missed menstrual periods, or repeated miscarriages —and male infertility
- symptoms involving the mouth, such as canker sores; a dry mouth; or a red, smooth, shiny tongue

Most people with celiac disease have one or more symptoms before they are diagnosed and begin treatment. Symptoms typically improve and may go away after a person begins eating a gluten-free diet. Symptoms may return if a person consumes small amounts of gluten.

Depending on how old you are when a doctor diagnoses your celiac disease, some symptoms, such as short height and tooth defects, may not improve. People with celiac disease who have no symptoms can still develop complications over time if they do not get treatment.

Dermatitis herpetiformis

Dermatitis herpetiformis is an itchy, blistering skin rash that usually appears on the elbows, knees, buttocks, back, or scalp. Among people with untreated celiac disease, about 2 to 3 percent of children and 10 to 20 percent of adults have dermatitis herpetiformis.[3] Some people with celiac disease may have the rash and no other symptoms. After a person starts a gluten-free diet, the rash may take some time to heal and may return if a person consumes small amounts of gluten.

What causes celiac disease?

Research suggests that celiac disease only occurs in people who have certain genes and eat food that contains gluten. Experts are studying other factors that may play a role in causing the disease.

Genes

Celiac disease almost always occurs in people who have one of two groups of normal gene variants, called DQ2 and DQ8. People who do not have these gene variants are very unlikely to develop celiac disease. About 30 percent of people have DQ2 or DQ8. However, only about 3 percent of people with DQ2 or DQ8 develop celiac disease.[4]

Researchers are studying other genes that may increase the chance of developing celiac disease in people who have DQ2 or DQ8.

Gluten

Consuming gluten triggers the abnormal immune system response that causes celiac disease. However, not all people who have the gene variants DQ2 or DQ8 and eat gluten develop the disease. Research suggests that among children with a genetic predisposition for celiac disease, those who eat more gluten in early childhood may have a greater risk for celiac disease.[5]

Other factors

Researchers are studying other factors that may increase a person's chances of developing celiac disease. For example, research suggest that a higher number of infections in early life and certain digestive tract infections may increase the risk. Experts also think changes in the microbiome—the bacteria in the digestive tract that help with digestion—could play a role in the development of celiac disease.

How do doctors diagnose celiac disease?

Doctors use information from your medical and family history, a physical exam, a dental exam, and medical test results to look for signs that you might have celiac disease and should be tested. Doctors typically diagnose celiac disease with blood tests and biopsies of the small intestine.

Medical and family history

Your doctor will ask about your symptoms. Celiac disease isn't diagnosed based on symptoms alone because some of the symptoms are like the symptoms of other digestive disorders, such as irritable bowel syndrome (IBS) or lactose intolerance. Some people with celiac disease have symptoms that affect parts of the body outside the digestive tract.

The doctor will review your medical history, including your history of conditions that are more common in people who have celiac disease. Your doctor will also ask about your family's medical history and whether anyone in your family has been diagnosed with celiac disease.

Physical exam

During a physical exam, a doctor may

- check for signs of weight loss or growth problems
- examine your skin for rashes, such as dermatitis herpetiformis
- listen to sounds in the abdomen using a stethoscope
- tap on the abdomen to check for pain or swelling

In some cases, a dentist may notice signs of celiac disease during an exam. Celiac disease may cause problems with the teeth and mouth, such as defects in tooth enamel or canker sores.

What tests do doctors use to diagnose celiac disease?

Doctors most often use blood tests and biopsies of the small intestine to diagnose or rule out celiac disease. Doctors don't recommend starting a gluten-free diet before diagnostic testing because a gluten-free diet can affect test results.

In some cases, doctors may order additional tests, such as skin biopsies and genetic tests, to help diagnose or rule out celiac disease.

Blood tests

A health care professional will take a blood sample from you and send the sample to a lab. Blood tests can show levels of certain antibodies that are often higher than normal in people who have untreated celiac disease. Blood tests may also show signs of health problems that could be related to celiac disease, such as anemia.

Biopsies of the small intestine

A doctor obtains biopsies of the small intestine during an upper GI endoscopy. For an upper GI endoscopy, a doctor uses an endoscope—a flexible tube with a camera—to see the lining of your upper GI tract, including the first part of your small intestine. The doctor passes an instrument through the endoscope to take small pieces of tissue from your small intestine. A pathologist will examine the tissue under a microscope to look for signs of celiac disease.

Skin biopsies

A doctor may order skin biopsies if you have a rash that could be dermatitis herpetiformis. For skin biopsies, a doctor removes small pieces of skin tissue on and next to the rash. A pathologist will examine the tissue under a microscope to look for signs of dermatitis herpetiformis.

Genetic testing

In some cases, a health care professional may take a blood sample or use a swab to collect cells from the inside of your cheek. The sample will be tested for groups of gene variants called DQ2 and DQ8. If you do not have these gene variants, you are very unlikely to have celiac disease.

Having DQ2 or DQ8 alone does not mean you have celiac disease. Most people with these gene variants do not develop celiac disease. If you do have DQ2 or DQ8, your doctor may recommend additional tests to check for or rule out celiac disease.

Do doctors screen for celiac disease?

Screening is testing for diseases when you have no symptoms. Doctors in the United States do not routinely screen people for celiac disease. However, blood relatives of people with celiac disease and those with type 1 diabetes should talk with their doctor about their chances of getting the disease to see if they should be tested.

How do doctors treat celiac disease?

Gluten-free diet

Doctors treat celiac disease by helping people to follow a gluten-free diet. Gluten is a protein found naturally in certain grains, including wheat, barley, and rye. Gluten is also added to many other foods and products. In people who have celiac disease, consuming gluten triggers an abnormal immune system reaction that damages the small intestine.

Symptoms greatly improve for most people with celiac disease who stick to a gluten-free diet. For most people, following a gluten-free diet will heal damage in the small intestine and prevent more damage. Many people see symptoms improve within days to weeks of starting the diet.[6]

Your doctor will explain the gluten-free diet and may refer you to a registered dietitian who specializes in treating people who have celiac disease. The dietitian will teach you how to avoid gluten while following a healthy diet and recommend substitutes for foods that contain gluten. He or she will help you

- check food and product labels for gluten
- design everyday meal plans
- make healthy choices about foods and drinks

Avoiding medicines and other products that may contain gluten

In addition to prescribing a gluten-free diet, your doctor will want you to avoid all hidden sources of gluten. If you have celiac disease, ask a pharmacist about ingredients in

- herbal and nutritional supplements
- prescription and over-the-counter medicines
- vitamin and mineral supplements

Medicines are rare sources of gluten. Even if gluten is present in a medicine, it is likely to be in such small quantities that it would not cause any symptoms.

Other products can be hidden sources of gluten. You may take in small amounts of gluten if you consume these products, use them around your mouth, or transfer them from your hands to your mouth by accident. Products that may contain gluten include

- children's modeling dough, such as Play-Doh
- cosmetics
- lipstick, lip gloss, and lip balm
- skin and hair products
- toothpaste and mouthwash
- communion wafers

Reading product labels can sometimes help you avoid gluten. Some companies label their products as being gluten-free. In the United States, products labelled gluten-free must have less than 20 parts per million of gluten, which should not be a problem for the vast majority of people. If a label doesn't tell you what is in a product, ask the company that makes the product for an ingredients list. You cannot assume that the product is gluten-free.

Treatments for symptoms or complications

A gluten-free diet will treat or prevent many of the symptoms and complications of celiac disease. Some symptoms may take longer to get better than others, and some symptoms may need additional help.

<u>Dermatitis herpetiformis</u> may not go away until a person has been following a gluten-free diet for 6 months to 2 years. In some cases, doctors may prescribe a medicine, such as <u>dapsone</u>, to help treat dermatitis herpetiformis until the rash is under control with a gluten-free diet alone.

In untreated celiac disease, damage to the small intestine can lead to <u>malabsorption</u> and malnutrition. When you are diagnosed with celiac disease, your doctor may test you for low levels of certain vitamins and minerals and may recommend or prescribe supplements if you need them. For safety reasons, talk with your doctor before using dietary supplements, such as vitamins, or any complementary or alternative medicines or medical practices.

When you are diagnosed with celiac disease, your doctor may recommend additional testing if you are at risk for certain complications. For example, doctors may order a bone mineral density test to check for osteoporosis.

Follow-up

Your doctor may recommend regular follow-up visits to make sure symptoms and health problems related to celiac disease are improving on a gluten-free diet. Follow-up may include blood tests to check levels of certain antibodies, which are higher in untreated celiac disease but typically return to normal after treatment. In some cases, doctors may recommend additional biopsies to find out if the small intestine has healed.

What if a gluten-free diet isn't working?

If you continue to have celiac disease symptoms while you are following a gluten-free diet, talk with your doctor or a registered dietitian, who can help you find the cause. In about 20 percent of people with celiac disease, symptoms continue or come back even while they are following a gluten-free diet.[7] Symptoms may be caused by consuming small amounts of gluten, other health problems, or refractory celiac disease.

Consuming small amounts of gluten

If your symptoms continue or come back after you start a gluten-free diet, you may still be eating or drinking a small amount of gluten. Keep a food journal and talk with your doctor and a registered dietitian about your diet and products you use that might contain gluten. Finding and avoiding all sources of gluten may help your symptoms improve. Hidden sources of gluten include additives made with wheat, such as

- modified food starch
- malt flavoring
- preservatives
- stabilizer

Other health problems

Your doctor may order tests to confirm the diagnosis of celiac disease and check for other health problems. Health problems that cause symptoms similar to those of celiac disease and may occur along with celiac disease include irritable bowel syndrome, lactose intolerance, microscopic colitis, problems with the pancreas, or small intestinal bacterial overgrowth.

Refractory celiac disease

Refractory celiac disease is a rare condition in which symptoms and damage to the small intestine continue or come back, even while a person is following a strict gluten-free diet. Refractory celiac disease may lead to complications, such as malnutrition or a type of cancer called enteropathy-associated T-cell lymphoma.

Doctors may recommend additional testing and treatments to diagnose and manage refractory celiac disease.

How will I need to change my diet if I have celiac disease?

If you have celiac disease, you will need to remove foods and drinks that contain gluten from your diet. Following a gluten-free diet can relieve celiac disease symptoms and heal damage to the small intestine. People with celiac disease need to follow a gluten-free diet for life to prevent symptoms and intestinal damage from coming back. Your doctor or a registered dietitian can guide you on what to eat and drink to maintain a balanced diet.

If you or your child has been diagnosed with celiac disease, you may find support groups helpful as you learn about and adjust to a gluten-free lifestyle. Your doctor or a registered dietitian may be able to recommend support groups and other reliable sources of information.

What foods and drinks contain gluten?

Gluten occurs naturally in certain grains, including

- wheat and types of wheat, such as durum, emmer, semolina, and spelt
- barley, which may be found in malt, malt extract, malt vinegar, and brewer's yeast
- rye
- triticale, a cross between wheat and rye

Gluten is found in foods that contain ingredients made from these grains, including baked goods, baking mixes, breads, cereals, and pastas. Drinks such as beer, lagers, ale, flavored liquors, and malt beverages may also contain gluten.

Many food ingredients and additives External link—such as colorings, flavorings, starches, and thickeners—are made from grains that contain gluten. These ingredients are added to many processed foods, including foods that are boxed, canned, frozen, packaged, or prepared. Therefore, gluten may be found in a variety of foods, including candy, condiments, hot dogs and sausages, ice cream, salad dressing, and soups.

Cross-contact

Cross-contact occurs when foods or products that contain gluten come into contact with gluten-free foods. Cross-contact can spread gluten to gluten-free foods, making the gluten-free foods unsafe for people with celiac disease to consume. Cross-contact can occur at any time, including when foods are grown, processed, stored, prepared, or served.

How can I identify and avoid foods and drinks that contain gluten?

A registered dietitian can help you learn to identify and avoid foods and drinks that contain gluten when you shop, prepare foods at home, or eat out.

For example, when you shop and eat at home

- carefully read food labels to check for grains that contain gluten—such as wheat, barley, and rye—and ingredients or additives made from those grains.
- check for gluten-free food labeling.
- don't eat foods if you aren't sure whether they contain gluten. If possible, contact the company that makes the food or visit the company's website for more information.

- store and prepare your gluten-free foods separately from other family members' foods that contain gluten to prevent cross-contact.

When you eat out at restaurants or social gatherings

- before you go out to eat, search online for restaurants that offer a gluten-free menu.
- review restaurant menus online or call ahead to make sure a restaurant can accommodate you safely.
- at the restaurant, let the server know that you have celiac disease. Ask about food ingredients, how food is prepared, and whether a gluten-free menu is available. Ask to talk with the chef if you would like more details about the menu.
- when attending social gatherings, let the host know you have celiac disease and find out if gluten-free foods will be available. If not, or if you are unsure, bring gluten-free foods that are safe for you to eat.

What should I eat if I have celiac disease?

If you have celiac disease, you will need to follow a gluten-free diet. Your doctor and a registered dietitian can help you plan a healthy, balanced diet to make sure that you get the nutrients you need.

Gluten-free foods

Many foods, such as meat, fish, fruits, vegetables, rice, and potatoes, without additives or some seasonings, are naturally gluten-free. Flour made from gluten-free foods, such as potatoes, rice, corn, soy, nuts, cassava, amaranth, quinoa, buckwheat, or beans are safe to eat.

You can also buy packaged gluten-free foods, such as gluten-free types of baked goods, bread, and pasta. These foods are available from many grocery stores, restaurants, and at specialty food companies. Packaged gluten-free foods tend to cost more than the same foods that have gluten, and restaurants may charge more for gluten-free types of foods.

Talk with your doctor or a registered dietitian about whether you should include oats in your diet and how much. Research suggests that most people with celiac disease can safely eat moderate amounts of oats. If you do eat oats, make sure they are gluten-free. Cross-contact between oats and grains that contain gluten is common and can make oats unsafe for people with celiac disease.

Gluten-free labeling

The U.S. Food and Drug Administration (FDA) requires that foods labeled "gluten-free" meet specific standards. One requirement is that foods with the terms "gluten-free," "no gluten," "free of gluten," or "without gluten" on the label must contain less than 20 parts per million of gluten. This amount of gluten is too small to cause problems in most people with celiac disease.

The FDA rule does not apply to foods regulated by the U.S. Department of Agriculture, including meat, poultry, and some egg products. The rule also does not apply to most alcoholic beverages, which are regulated by the U.S. Department of the Treasury.

Should I start a gluten-free diet before I talk with my doctor?

No. If you think you might have celiac disease, you should talk with your doctor about testing to diagnose celiac disease before you begin a gluten-free diet. If you avoid gluten before you have testing, the test results may not be accurate.

Also, if you start avoiding gluten without advice from a doctor or a registered dietitian, your diet may not provide enough of the nutrients you need, such as fiber, iron, and calcium. Some packaged gluten-free foods may be higher in fat and sugar than the same foods that contain gluten. If you are diagnosed with celiac disease, your doctor and dietitian can help you plan a healthy gluten-free diet.

If you don't have celiac disease or another health problem related to gluten, your doctor may not recommend a gluten-free diet. In recent years, more people without celiac disease have begun avoiding gluten, believing that a gluten-free diet is healthier or could help them lose weight. However, researchers have found no evidence that a gluten-free diet promotes better health or weight loss for the general population.

Appendix A: Guide to Better Living

Note: Always consult your physician before making any changes to your diet, physical activity or life style.

Is your health condition requires that you make changes to your diet, physical activity, or life style? Are you thinking about being more active? Have you been trying to cut back on less healthy foods? Are you starting to eat better and move more but having a hard time sticking with these changes?

Old habits die hard. Changing your habits is a process that involves several stages. Sometimes it takes a while before changes become new habits. And, you may face roadblocks along the way.

Adopting new, healthier habits may protect you from serious health problems. New habits, like healthy eating and regular physical activity, may also help you manage your weight and have more energy. After a while, if you stick with these changes, they may become part of your daily routine.

The information below outlines four stages you may go through when changing your health habits or behavior. You will also find tips to help you improve your eating, physical activity habits, and overall health. The four stages of changing a health behavior are

- contemplation
- preparation
- action
- maintenance

What stage of change are you in?

Contemplation: "I'm thinking about it."

In this first stage, you are thinking about change and becoming motivated to get started.

You might be in this stage if you

- have been considering change but are not quite ready to start
- believe that your health, energy level, or overall well-being will improve if you develop new habits
- are not sure how you will overcome the roadblocks that may keep you from starting to change

Preparation: "I have made up my mind to take action."

In this next stage, you are making plans and

thinking of specific ideas that will work for you.

You might be in this stage if you

- have decided that you are going to change and are ready to take action
- have set some specific goals that you would like to meet
- are getting ready to put your plan into action

Action: "I have started to make changes."

In this third stage, you are acting on your plan and making the changes you set out to achieve.

You might be in this stage if you

- have been making eating, physical activity, and other behavior changes in the last 6 months or so
- are adjusting to how it feels to eat healthier, be more active, and make other changes such as getting more sleep or reducing screen time
- have been trying to overcome things that sometimes block your success

Maintenance: "I have a new routine."

In this final stage, you have become used to your changes and have kept them up for more than 6 months.

You might be in this stage if

- your changes have become a normal part of your routine
- you have found creative ways to stick with your routine
- you have had slip-ups and setbacks but have been able to get past them and make progress

Did you find your stage of change? Read on for ideas about what you can do next.

Contemplation: Are you thinking of making changes?

Making the leap from thinking about change to taking action can be hard and may take time. Asking yourself about the pros (benefits) and cons (things that get in the way) of changing your habits may be helpful. How would life be better if you made some changes?

Think about how the benefits of healthy eating or regular physical activity might relate to your overall health. For example, suppose your blood glucose, also called blood sugar, is a bit high and you have a parent, brother, or sister who has type 2 diabetes. This means you also may develop type 2 diabetes. You may find that it is easier to be physically active and eat healthy knowing that it may help control blood glucose and protect you from a serious disease.

You may learn more about the benefits of changing your eating and physical activity habits from a health care professional. This knowledge may help you take action.

Look at the lists of pros and cons below. Find the items you believe are true for you. Think about factors that are important to you.

Healthy Eating

Pros
- have more energy
- improve my health
- lower my risk for health problems
- maintain a healthy weight
- feel proud of myself
- set an example for friends and family

Cons
- may spend more money and time on food
- may need to cook more often at home
- may need to eat less of foods I love
- may need to buy different foods
- may need to convince my family that we all have to eat healthier foods

Physical Activity

Pros

- improve my health
- reduce my risk for serious health problems
- feel better about myself
- become stronger
- have fun
- take time to care for myself
- meet new people and spend time with them
- have more energy
- maintain a healthy weight
- become a role model for others

Cons

- takes too much time and energy
- it is too hot or cold outside
- feel self-conscious
- am nervous about my health
- could hurt myself
- am not good at being active
- do not know what to do
- have no one to be active with
- am not young or fit enough
- keeps me from family and friends

Preparation: Have you made up your mind?

If you are in the preparation stage, you are about to take action. To get started, look at your list of pros and cons. How can you make a plan and act on it?

The chart below lists common roadblocks you may face and possible solutions to overcome roadblocks as you begin to change your habits. Think about these things as you make your plan.

Roadblock: I don't have time.

Solution: Make your new healthy habit a priority. Fit in physical activity whenever and wherever you can. Try taking the stairs or getting off the bus a stop early if it is safe to do so. Set aside one grocery shopping day a week, and make healthy meals that you can freeze and eat later when you don't have time to cook.

Roadblock: Healthy habits cost too much.

Solution: You can walk around the mall, a school track, or a local park for free. Eat healthy on a budget by buying in bulk and when items are on sale, and by choosing frozen or canned fruits and vegetables.

Roadblock: I can't make this change alone.

Solution: Recruit others to be active with you, which will help you stay motivated and safe. Consider signing up for a fun fitness class like salsa dancing. Get your family or coworkers on the healthy eating bandwagon. Plan healthy meals together with your family, or start a healthy potluck once a week at work.

Roadblock: I don't like physical activity.

Solution: Forget the old notion that being physically active means lifting weights in a gym. You can be active in many ways, including dancing, walking, or gardening. Make your own list of options that appeal to you. Explore options you never thought about, and stick with what you enjoy.

Roadblock: I don't like healthy foods.

Solution: Try making your old favorite recipes in healthier new ways. For example, you can trim fat from meats and reduce the amount of butter, sugar, and salt you cook with. Use low-fat cheeses or milk rather than whole-milk foods. Add a cup or two of broccoli, carrots, or spinach to casseroles or pasta.

Once you have made up your mind to change your habits, make a plan and set goals for taking action. Here are some ideas for making your plan:

- learn more about healthy eating (https://www.myplate.gov/)
- learn more about being active (see appendix B)
- make lists of
  - healthy foods that you like or may need to eat more of—or more often
  - foods you love that you may need to eat less often
  - things you could do to be more physically active
  - fun activities you like and could do more often, such as dancing

After making your plan, start setting goals for putting your plan into action. Start with small changes. For example, "I'm going to walk for 10 minutes, three times a week." What is the one step you can take right away?

Action: Have you started to make changes?

You are making real changes to your lifestyle, which is fantastic! To stick with your new habits

- review your plan
- look at the goals you set and how well you are meeting them
- overcome roadblocks by planning ahead for setbacks
- reward yourself for your hard work

Track your progress

- Tracking your progress helps you spot your strengths, find areas where you can improve, and stay on course. Record not only what you did, but how you felt while doing it—your feelings can play a role in making your new habits stick.

- Recording your progress may help you stay focused and catch setbacks in meeting your goals. Remember that a setback does not mean you have failed. All of us experience setbacks. The key is to get back on track as soon as you can.

- You can track your progress with online tools such as the NIH Body Weight Planner (https://www.youtube.com/watch?v=v1gluQwi eog). The NIH Body Weight Planner lets you tailor your calorie and physical activity plans to reach your personal goals within a specific time period.

Overcome roadblocks

- Remind yourself why you want to be healthier. Perhaps you want the energy to play with your nieces and nephews or to be able to carry your own grocery bags. Recall your reasons for making changes when slip-ups occur. Decide to take the first step to get back on track.

- Problem-solve to "outsmart" roadblocks. For example, plan to walk indoors, such as at a mall, on days when bad weather keeps you from walking outside.
- Ask a friend or family member for help when you need it, and always try to plan ahead. For example, if you know that you will not have time to be physically active after work, go walking with a coworker at lunch or start your day with an exercise video.

Reward yourself

- After reaching a goal or milestone, allow for a nonfood reward such as new workout gear or a new workout device. Also consider posting a message on social media to share your success with friends and family.
- Choose rewards carefully. Although you should be proud of your progress, keep in mind that a high-calorie treat or a day off from your activity routine are not the best rewards to keep you healthy.
- Pat yourself on the back. When negative thoughts creep in, remind yourself how much good you are doing for your health by moving more and eating healthier.

Maintenance: Have you created a new routine?

Make your future a healthy one. Remember that eating healthy, getting regular physical activity, and other healthy habits are lifelong behaviors, not one-time events. Always keep an eye on your efforts and seek ways to deal with the planned and unplanned changes in life.

Now that healthy eating and regular physical activity are part of your routine, keep things interesting, avoid slip-ups, and find ways to cope with what life throws at you.

Add variety and stay motivated

Mix up your routine with new physical activities and goals, physical activity buddies, foods, recipes, and rewards.

Deal with unexpected setbacks

Plan ahead to avoid setbacks. For example, find other ways to be active in case of bad weather, injury, or other issues that arise. Think of ways to eat healthy when traveling or dining out, like packing healthy snacks while on the road or sharing an entrée with a friend in a restaurant.

If you do have a setback, don't give up. Setbacks happen to everyone. Regroup and focus on meeting your goals again as soon as you can.

Challenge yourself!

Revisit your goals and think of ways to expand them. For example, if you are comfortable walking 5 days a week, consider adding strength training twice a week. If you have limited your saturated fat intake by eating less fried foods, try cutting back on added sugars, too. Small changes can lead to healthy habits worth keeping.

**When The Going Gets Tough,
Put One Foot in Front of The
Other and Just Keep Going.
Don't Give Up!**

Appendix B: How to Stay Active

Note: Always consult your physician before making any changes to your diet, physical activity or life style.

Physical activity may seem hard if you're overweight. You may get short of breath or tired quickly. Finding or affording the right clothes and equipment may be frustrating. Or, perhaps you may not feel comfortable working out in front of others.

The good news is you can overcome these challenges. Not only can you be active at any size, you can have fun and feel good at the same time.

Can anyone be active?

Research strongly shows that physical activity is safe for almost everyone. The health benefits of physical activity far outweigh the risks.

The activities discussed here are safe for most people. If you have problems moving or staying steady on your feet, or if you get out of breath easily, talk with a health care professional before you start. You also should talk with a health care professional if you are unsure of your health, have any concerns that physical activity may be unsafe for you, or have

- a chronic disease such as diabetes, high blood pressure, or heart disease
- a bone or joint problem—for example, in your back, knee, or hip—that could get worse if you change your physical activity level

Why should I be active?

Being active may help you live longer and protect you from developing serious health problems, such as type 2 diabetes, heart disease, stroke, and certain types of cancer. Regular physical activity is linked to many health benefits, such as

- lower blood pressure and blood glucose, or blood sugar
- healthy bones, muscles, and joints
- a strong heart and lungs
- better sleep at night and improved mood

The Physical Activity Guidelines for Americans define regular physical activity as at least 150 minutes a week of moderate-intensity aerobic activity, such as brisk walking. Brisk walking is a pace of 3 miles per hour or faster. A moderate-intensity activity makes you breathe harder but does not overwork or overheat you. You should also do muscle-strengthening activities at least 2 days a week.

You may reach this goal by starting with 5 minutes

of physical activity several times a day, 5 to 6 days a week. You could then gradually work up to 10 minutes per session, 3 times a day. If you do even more activity, you may gain even more health benefits.

When combined with healthy eating, regular physical activity may also help you control your weight. However, research shows that even if you can't lose weight or maintain your weight loss, you still can enjoy important health benefits from regular physical activity.

Physical activity also can be a lot of fun if you do activities you enjoy and are active with other people. Being active with others may give you a chance to meet new people or spend more time with family and friends. You also may inspire and motivate one another to get and stay active.

What do I need to know about becoming active?

Choosing physical activities that match your fitness level and health goals can help you stay motivated and keep you from getting hurt. You may feel some minor discomfort or muscle soreness when you first become active. These feelings should go away as you get used to your activity. However, if you feel sick to your stomach or have pain, you may have done too much. Go easier and then slowly build up your activity level. Some activities, such as walking or swimming, are less likely to cause injuries.

If you have been inactive, start slowly and see how you feel. Gradually increase how long and how often you are active. If you need guidance, check with a health care or certified fitness professional.

Here are some tips for staying safe during physical activity:

- Wear the proper safety gear, such as a bike helmet if you are bicycling.
- Make sure any sports equipment you use works and fits properly.
- Look for safe places to be active. For instance, walk in well-lit areas where other people are around. Be active with a friend or group.
- Stay hydrated to replace the body fluids you lose through sweating and to prevent you from getting overheated.
- If you are active outdoors, protect yourself from the sun with sunscreen and a hat or protective visor and clothing.
- Wear enough clothing to keep warm in cold or windy weather. Layers are best.

If you don't feel right, stop your activity. If you have any of the following warning signs, stop and seek help right away:

- pain, tightness, or pressure in your chest or neck, shoulder, or arm
- extreme shortness of breath
- dizziness or sickness

Check with a health care professional about what to do if you have any of these warning signs. If your activity is causing pain in your joints, feet, ankles, or legs, you also should consult a health care professional to see if you may need to change the type or amount of activity you are doing.

What kinds of activities can I do?

You don't need to be an athlete or have special skills or equipment to make physical activity part of your life. Many types of activities you do every day, such as walking your dog or going up and down steps at home or at work, may help improve your health.

Try different activities you enjoy. If you like an activity, you're more likely to stick with it. Anything that gets you moving around, even for a few minutes at a time, is a healthy start to getting fit.

Walking

Walking is free and easy to do—and you can do it

almost anywhere. Walking will help you

- burn calories
- improve your fitness
- lift your mood
- strengthen your bones and muscles

If you are concerned about safety, try walking in a shopping mall or park where it is well lit and other people are around. Many malls and parks have benches where you can take a quick break. Walking with a friend or family member is safer than walking alone and may provide the social support you need to meet your activity goals.

If you don't have time for a long walk, take several short walks instead. For example, instead of a 30-minute walk, add three 10-minute walks to your day. Shorter spurts of activity are easier to fit into a busy schedule.

Walking tips

- Wear comfortable, well-fitting walking shoes with a lot of support, and socks that absorb sweat.
- Dress for the weather if you are walking outdoors. In cold weather, wear layers of clothing you can remove if you start getting too warm. In hot weather, protect yourself against the sun and heat.

- Warm up by walking more slowly for the first few minutes. Cool down by slowing your pace.

Dancing

Dancing can be a lot of fun while it tones your muscles, strengthens your heart and lungs, and boosts your mood. You can dance at a health club, dance studio, or even at home. Just turn on some lively music and start moving. You also can dance to a video on your TV or computer.

If you have trouble standing on your feet for a long time, try dancing while sitting down. Chair dancing lets you move your arms and legs to music while taking the weight off your feet.

Bicycling

Riding a bicycle spreads your weight among your arms, back, and hips. For outdoor biking, you may want to try a mountain bike. Mountain bikes have wider tires and are sturdier than bikes with thinner tires. You can buy a larger seat to make biking more comfortable.

For indoor biking, you may want to try a recumbent bike. On this type of bike, you sit lower to the ground with your legs reaching forward to the pedals. Your body is in more of a reclining position, which may feel better than sitting straight up. The seat on a recumbent bike is also wider than the seat on a regular bike.

If you decide to buy a bike, check how much weight it can support to make sure it is safe for you.

Workout clothing tips

- Clothes made of fabrics that absorb sweat are best for working out.
- Comfortable, lightweight clothes allow you to move more easily.
- Tights or spandex shorts are the best bottoms to wear to prevent inner-thigh chafing.
- Women should wear a bra that provides extra support during physical activity.

Water workouts

Swimming and water workouts put less stress on your joints than walking, dancing, or biking. If your feet, back, or joints hurt when you stand, water activities may be best for you. If you feel self-conscious about wearing a bathing suit, you can wear shorts and a T-shirt while you swim.

Exercising in water

- Lets you be more flexible. You can move your body in water in ways you may not be able to on land.

- Reduces your risk of hurting yourself. Water provides a natural cushion, which keeps you from pounding or jarring your joints.
- Helps prevent sore muscles.
- Keeps you cool, even when you are working hard.

You don't need to know how to swim to work out in water. You can do shallow- or deep-water exercises at either end of the pool without swimming. For instance, you can do laps while holding onto a kickboard and kicking your feet. You also can walk or jog across the width of the pool while moving your arms.

For shallow-water workouts, the water level should be between your waist and chest. During deep-water workouts, most of your body is underwater. For safety and comfort, wear a foam belt or life jacket.

Tips for protecting your hair

If you're worried that pool water will damage or mess up your hair, try these tips:

- Use a swim cap to help protect your hair from pool chemicals and getting wet.
- Wear a natural hairstyle, short braids, locs, or twists, which may be easier to style after a water workout.

- Buy a shampoo to remove chlorine buildup, available at most drug stores, if your hair feels dry or damaged after a pool workout.

Strength training

Strength training involves using free weights, weightlifting machines, resistance bands, or your own body weight to make your muscles stronger. Lower-body strength training will improve your balance and prevent falls.

Strength training may help you

- build and maintain strong muscles as you get older
- continue to perform activities of daily living, such as carrying groceries or moving furniture
- keep your bones strong, which may help prevent osteoporosis and fractures

If you are just starting out, using a weightlifting machine may be safer than dumbbells. As you get fit, you may want to add free-weight exercises with dumbbells.

You do not need a weight bench or large dumbbells to do strength training at home. You can use a pair of hand weights to do bicep curls. You can also use your own body weight: for example, get up and down from a chair.

Proper form is very important when lifting weights. You may hurt yourself if you don't lift weights properly. You may want to schedule a session with a certified fitness professional to learn which exercises to do and how to do them safely. Check with your health insurer about whether your health plan covers these services.

If you decide to buy a home gym, check how much weight it can support to make sure it is safe for you.

Strength-training tips

- Aim for at least 2 days per week of strengthen-training activities.
- Try to perform each exercise 8 to 12 times. If that's too hard, the weight you are lifting is too heavy. If it's too easy, your weight is too light.
- Try to exercise all the major muscle groups. These groups include the muscles of the legs, hips, chest, back, abdomen, shoulders, and arms.
- Don't work the same muscles 2 days in a row. Your muscles need time to recover.

Mind and body exercise

Your local hospital or fitness, recreation, or community center may offer classes such as yoga, tai chi, or Pilates. You also may find some of these workouts online and can download them to a computer, smart phone, or other device. These types of activities may help you

- become stronger and more flexible
- feel more relaxed
- improve balance and posture

Your local hospital or fitness, recreation, or community center may offer classes such as yoga, tai chi, or Pilates.

These classes also can be a lot of fun and add variety to your workout routine. If some movements are hard to do or you have injuries you are concerned about, talk with the instructor about how to adapt the exercises and poses to meet your needs—or start with a beginner's class.

Daily life activities

Daily life activities, such as cleaning out the attic or washing the car, are great ways to get moving. Small changes can add more physical activity to your day and improve your health. Try these:

- Take 2- to 3-minute walking breaks at work several times a day, if possible.
- Stand, walk, or stretch in place during TV commercials.
- Take the stairs instead of the elevator or escalator whenever you can.

- Park farther from where you are going and walk the rest of the way.

Even a shopping trip can be exercise because it provides a chance to walk and carry your bags. Chores such as mowing the lawn, raking leaves, and gardening also count.

Where can I be active?

You can find many fun places to be active. Having more than one place may keep you from getting bored. Here are some options:

- Join or take a class at a local fitness, recreation, or community center.
- Enjoy the outdoors by taking a hike or going for a walk in a safe local park, neighborhood, or mall.
- Work out in the comfort of your own home with a workout video or by finding a fitness channel on your TV, tablet, or other mobile device.

Tips for choosing a fitness center

- Make sure the center has exercise equipment for people who weigh more and staff to show you how to use it.
- Ask if the center has any special classes for people just starting out, older adults, or people with mobility or health issues.

- See if you can try out the center or take a class before you join.
- Try to find a center close to work or home. The quicker and easier the center is to get to, the better your chances of using it often.
- Make sure you understand the rules for joining and ending your membership, what your membership fee covers, any related costs, and the days and hours of operation.

How can I get past my roadblocks?

You most likely will face roadblocks that keep you from meeting your physical activity goals. Think about what keeps you from being active, then try to come up with creative ways to address those roadblocks. Here are a few examples to help you get started:

Barrier: I don't have enough time.

Solution: Instead of doing one long workout session, build in three 10-minute bursts of activity during your day, such as a brisk walk. Even standing up instead of sitting at your desk has benefits.

Barrier: I just don't like exercise.

Solution: Good news! You don't have to run a marathon or go to the gym all the time to benefit from being active. To make physical activity more fun, try something you enjoy doing, such as dancing to the radio or taking a yoga class with friends. Many people find they start to like exercise better the more they do it.

Barrier: I'm worried about my health or getting hurt.

Solution: If you have a hard time being active because of your health, talk with a health care professional first. A certified fitness professional can also guide you on how to be active safely.

Barrier: I feel self-conscious working out in front of others.

Solution: Start being active at home until you feel more confident. Be active with friends who will support and encourage you.

How can I stick with my physical activity plan?

Sticking with a plan to be physically active can be a challenge. Online tools such as the NIH Body Weight Planner (https://www.youtube.com/watch?v=v1gluQwieog) can help. The NIH Body Weight Planner lets you tailor your calorie and physical activity plans to reach your personal goals within a specific time period.

You also can download fitness apps that let you enter information to track your progress using a computer or smart phone or other mobile device.

Devices you can wear, such as pedometers and fitness trackers, may help you count steps, calories, and minutes of physical activity. Trackers can help you set goals and monitor progress. You wear most of these devices on your wrist like a watch, or clipped to your clothing.

Keeping an activity journal is another good way to help you stay motivated and on track to reach your fitness goals.

Set goals. As you track your activity, try to set specific short- and long-term goals. For example, instead of "I will be more active," set a goal such as "I will take a walk after lunch at least 2 days a week." Getting started with a doable goal is a good way to form a new habit. A short-term goal may be to walk 5 to 10 minutes, 5 days a week. A long-term goal may be to do at least 150 minutes of moderate-intensity physical activity a week.

Get support. Ask a family member or friend to be active with you. Your workout buddy can help make your activities more fun and can cheer you on and help you meet your goals.

Track progress. You may not feel as though you

are making progress, but when you look back at where you started, you may be pleasantly surprised. Making regular activity part of your life is a big step. Start slowly and praise yourself for every goal you set and achieve.

Review your goals. Did you meet your goals? If not, why? Are they doable? Did you hit a roadblock trying to meet your goal? What will you do differently next week? Brainstorm some options to overcome future roadblocks. Ask a friend or family member to help support your goals.

Pick nonfood rewards. Whether your goal is to be active 15 minutes a day, to walk farther than you did last week, or simply to stay positive, recognizing your efforts is an important part of staying on track. Decide how you will reward yourself. Some ideas for rewards include getting new music to charge you up or buying new workout gear.

Be patient with yourself. Don't get discouraged if you have setbacks from time to time. If you can't achieve your goal the first time or can only stick to your goals for part of the week, remind yourself that this is all part of establishing new habits.

Look ahead. Try to focus on what you will do differently moving forward, rather than on what went wrong. Pat yourself on the back for trying.

Most importantly, don't give up. Any movement, even for a short time, is a good thing. Each activity you add to your life is another step toward a healthier you.

www.ingramcontent.com/pod-product-compliance
Lightning Source LLC
Chambersburg PA
CBHW070321160726
47999CB00003B/1099